Medicinal Herbs

Homemade Healing Remedies with 30 Herbs

Table of Contents

Introduction

I would first like to thank and congratulate you on downloading **"Medicinal Herbs: 30 Herbs and Herbal Blend Healing Remedies."** Herbal remedies are certainly not new they have been around for generations, the father of medicine, Hippocrates, was a great supporter of herbal therapy, even setting up his very own herbal clinics, at that was in 400BC!

Hippocrates always praised the wonderful healing herbs during his entire practice. One of his most famous quotes was "Nature Cures, not the Physician." Hippocrates was well aware that the healing herbs were powerful in treatments for many ailments.

Choosing natural remedies is a much healthier choice when compared to taking chemical filled synthetic drugs as forms of treatment. Mind you there are certain ailments that need synthetic drugs to treat them. I do not suggest taking any new form of treatment of a health issue or ailment until you have discussed it with your physician.

Many of us understand the power behind herbal roots, leaves of medicinal plants that are eaten whole or ground up to make a powder to used to make teas or added to our foods.

People that engage in naturopathy (healing from nature) tend to develop a distinctive philosophy and a positive can-do attitude when dealing with illness and disease. They respect and appreciate the herbal remedies that nature provides for us for free.

Using herbs for healing is something that is used all around the world, shared by all of humanity. People from all different parts of the world, with different cultures and beliefs will come together and agree on the affects that natural herbal medicine can have on treating our ailments.

The physicians throughout history have been well aware of the wonderful and tremendous resources we have in herbal remedies using roots, fruits, and flowers of medicinal plants in treating our ailments.

People are looking to find more healthier and natural approaches to living a healthy lifestyle which includes using more natural solutions to our daily aches and pains that we endure in life to more serious health issues such as cancer and diabetes.

In this book we will take a look at various medicinal herbs and what they can be good for treating and even curing without you having to suffer through severe side effects as well as you would if you were taking a synthetic treatment. Once you begin choosing more natural and healthy choices in your life from what you eat to what you are taking to treat health issues you are going to see a difference in your overall outlook and approach to life—it will become energized and positive, leaving you feeling content and stress free!

Chapter 1. Medicinal Herbs to Treat Your Aches and Pains

Because more people are getting more educated and realizing the harm that they are causing their bodies by feeding on synthetic and unnatural substances with bad side affects they are turning more and more to natural solutions to their aches and pains. Many modern treatments are becoming incredibly expensive and for many people that do not have some kind of health coverage they simply cannot afford to use modern methods of treatment.

However, with this being said we are also finding out that not only is medicinal medicine a more affordable choice for many but it is in fact considered by more and more people to be the safest and healthiest choice as a form of treatment for our various ailments.

When you sit down and really think about it what would seem to you the more healthy choice—the synthetic drug with severe side effects or the natural medicinal herbal treatment? I myself lean towards taking the natural choice as a form of treatment.

If you get the thumbs up from your physician to try the natural remedy for your ailment then why not give it a try all you may have to lose is not suffering from nasty side effects as well as putting foreign substances into your body that are made of unnatural ingredients. This in itself should have you sitting wondering how good can these foreign substances really be for my health in the long run?

Many of us suffer daily from aches and pains the technical term is 'Myalgia' which basically is translated to mean 'pain in the muscles.' One of these pains that is most common is called 'Fibromyalgia.' This is a very devastating disorder that involves the musculoskeletal system, followed by wide spread pain in the body that is accompanied with deep fatigue.

Some look at Fibromyalgia as the mother load of all aches and pains, it is caused by the imbalance of chemicals that causes a disruption which when the brain processes the signals it relates to them as pain signals. The good news is that there are medicinal herbs that can help treat this painful ailment and even possibly reverse it all together.

Using medicinal herbs can help to readjust and refine those pain processors of the brain, this will in turn allow you to rework how your body is interpreting external stressors. As our bodies age Fibromyalgia is just a magnification of the discomfort our bodies face the older we get. It is a deep rooted pain that is in our muscle tissue that can lead to much discomfort especially as our bodies age.

The human body is basically like a machine that with prolonged use it begins to wear out. But with some healthy herbs thrown into the mix these can really help to combat whatever it is that ails. Let us take a look at some healthy organic aids that can help you combat your aches and pains in life.

Turmeric. If you are someone that suffers from arthritis you may just have a new best friend in Turmeric. Turmeric will function much the same as Ginger does in that it acts as an inflammation reducer. Turmeric contains properties that have anti-inflammatory reactions that will ease into your aching wrists and joints. History shows a long use of Turmeric. Using

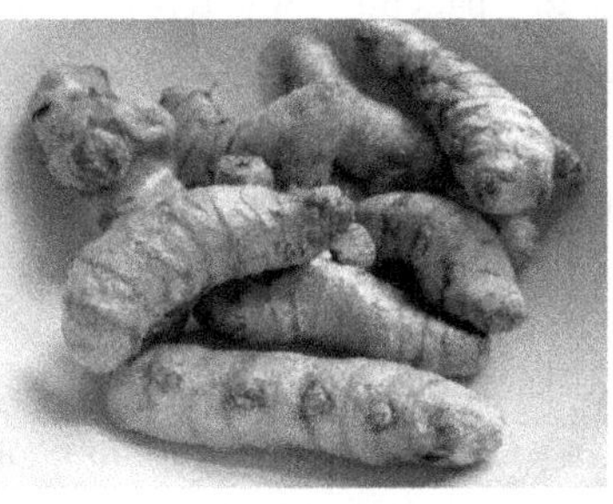

Turmeric can help you to lessen the pain of your arthritis and even eliminate it all together. You can also use it to help reduce heartburn, so you can use it to treat a backache or stomachache. It is also a very tasty seasoning to add to your meals such as chicken.

Devils Claw.   The name of this particular herb may not be appealing to many, but it does offer some wonderful healing properties despite its name.   For many generations devils claw has been used in the treatment of aches and pains.

It is especially promising when it comes to helping to treat back pain. The reason for this is that when devils claw is ground up into powder and applied in a compress to the lower back it can provide you with great relief of your back pain.

It originates from South Africa, this herb is sought out from many who suffer from back pain and want to avoid a trip to the chiropractor. There is documented research to back this up. In 2002 there was 227 patients that had been administered devils claw to treat back and hip pain.

Out of the 227 patients it was reported that 70% of them reported improvement and even an increase in mobility. This medicinal herb has the ability to loosen up the most stubborn of joints and muscles to help relieve your aches and pains. You can find devils claw at your local health food stores, it can also be grown as well.

Ginger. Using ginger extract has proven to give relief for most joint and muscle pain. The ginger will help to lessen the inflammation. You can grind the ginger into a powder and rub it into your aching joints to gain instant relief. You may also choose to make a tea and drink it.

Valerian Root. There is a long list of benefits connected to the Valerian root, one of the least known benefits is that it can help to relieve leg cramps and painful muscle spasms. Just apply it directly to your skin and allow the soothing to kick in.

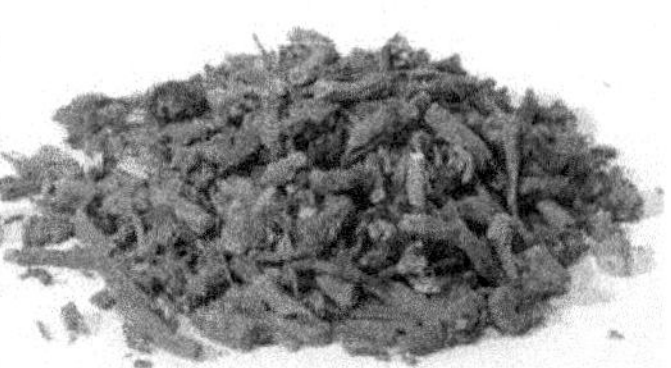

It has been shown in studies that this herb can work directly on the nervous system as a pain reliever. Valerian root is very popular for a wide number of reasons that surround musculoskeletal problems.

It is widely grown found in large amounts in areas such as Mexico, India, and Europe. Most often it is ground into a powder form, extracting the essential oil from the root, or boiled to be used as a beverage. I find that I enjoy making a nice tea with it to help ease my aching muscles from a hectic busy day.

Burdock Root. The Burdock Root is dry and oily that is well known for lubricating and moistening stiff joints. It is best to use when it is ground into a fine paste or powder and it is applied directly to the area where you are having the most aches and pains.

The flowers of the plant are usually either pink or purple and form into cluster and can grow to be 2 meters in height. You can find Burdock scattered around northern climates all across the globe it is most prevalent in late Spring and early Summer.

You can grind up the root of the Burdock plant and apply it to your joints or you can extract liquid by boiling it. The essential oil that is extracted from Burdock is very potent so you might want to mix it first with a base oil such as olive oil before you apply it.

Chapter 2. Give Your Immune System a Boost by Using Medicinal Herbs

Without our immune system we could not step out into the world beyond our front door, so it is very important in our survival. If we did not have it we would have to live in a bubble to protect ourselves from contaminates.

Included in your immune system is an army of white blood cells that fight against harmful bacteria and viruses on a daily basis. Your body will produce around 1000 white blood cells a day. The specialized part of your white blood cell army is called 'Macrophages' these go seek out any germs that may enter your system and once they locate them they destroy them.

We remain healthy largely due to our immune system being able to filter and eliminate harmful elements. It is good to give our immune system a little jumpstart once and a while. There are many herbs that can help you to achieve this.

Reishi.	The Reishi mushroom has been used in Chinese herbal medicine for thousands of years. This herb has been shown to improve the immune system while also improving longevity as well.

It has heavy antioxidant properties that have been used in the treatment of many ailments such as cancer and urinary infections.

This mushroom has been referred to as the 'immune modulator' for its magical properties that help to fine tune and regulate your immune system.

There is no special preparation needed all you need to do is eat it. When you regularly consume this mushroom you will see improvements in no time. It will help improve your blood flow and your overall immune health.

Echinachea.   Euchinachea is a member of the daisy family, it has great anti-biotic and anti-viral properties. Many people like to make a herbal tea and tonic from its extracted oil and use it to help give their immune system a boost to help in fighting off viruses, germs, and bacteria.

You can open your nasal passages with the aroma of this plant. Using moderate doses of this herb can help in the treatment of the worst cold and allergy symptoms. It can also aide with upper respiratory tract infections.

Astragalus. This is another Chinese herb that is been used by the Chinese for thousands of years as a herbal medicine. It is used today as a powerful immune booster. Many people take it in the form of a broth such as chicken broth. Using Astragalus in your soup is so powerful that it is known to directly activate the marrow of your lymph tissue and will stimulate the development of your active immune cells.

You can ground up the roots into powder and oil can be extracted to use in aroma therapy or it can be made into soothing creams for herbal massage. You can also use the leaves of this plant to make teas that will help the throat and empower the rest of your bodily functions. It is a very impressive herb and will be well worth the efforts of you obtaining it.

Cats Claw. The woodsy vine of cats claw is native to the rain forests of the Amazon in South America. It is very similar to Devils claw, it gets its name due to the curved claw shaped thorns that have a cat-like appearance to them. The cats claw roots have been used for thousands of years by the indigenous tribes in South America for healing and immune boosting properties that it offers. When you use this properly it can boost the white blood cell count in your system as well as regulate it.

Cats claw is recommended as an alternative treatment for Cancer and Aids. It is known to help in easing the harshness of chemotherapy for Cancer patients. It is often served in a tea or ground into powder that can be rubbed into your skin.

Chapter 3. Using Medicinal Herbs to Treat Anxiety and Depression

We are living in a fast paced world often rushing and stressing in our daily lives causes us to leave our peace of mind behind. Living in a way that is healthy both mentally and physically is not always done. As a result of this many of us will suffer from anxiety and depression. Here are some natural aids to help you to deal with your anxiety and depression that you are suffering from.

Lavender. Lavender is a great herb that has proven over time to be very effective in fighting against anxiety. The nice thing with this treatment is it will not have the side effect of making you sleepy.

You can take this herbal medicine at all hours throughout the day. You can apply it directly to your skin in the form of an essential oil allowing the aromatic healing and stress relief to take effect on you.

Ashwagandha. This is a medicinal herb that has proven to be a very powerful part of Ayurvedic medicine for many centuries. This is known to help the body to adapt to stressful situations. The roots of this plant will have a powerful effect on stress you may be feeling and will help to gently sooth the body and mind. The best way you can take this herb is to boil it and make a tea and drink it.

Kava. The Kava herb will help act as a mild sedative and will relax your body without disrupting the cognitive function, this allows you to relax without losing control of your everyday routine. Kava does not have any addictive properties so you can easily discontinue its use. It can cause liver damage with long time use and it has been banned in Europe. It is still available in most health food stores within the United States.

Passion Flower. This particular herb has been known to work just as well as many of the pharmaceutical prescribed anxiety medications. It has been able to heal depression, anxiety and irritability.

Lemon Balm. The Lemon Balm herb is from the mint family, it has been know to give a person the sense of calmness up to six hours. It was used in the middle-ages as a tonic to help in reducing stress. It was commonly used in medieval times as a medicine, food and even used in alcoholic drinks.

It can often been found combined with Chamomile and boiled in teas and other soothing hot drinks. Most of the medicinal aspect of this plant comes from its leaves. You can apply the leaves directly to your skin or you may choose to reduce them to a powder form and add to your bath water.

It is a herb that is native to Europe but you can find it growing just about any where in the world today. The Lemon Balm plant will grow to be about two feet in height and it is easily recognizable by its lovely bright yellow flowers.

Saffron. The Saffron plant itself does not look to special but it is well known in fighting against depression. It comes from the Iris family and is found all over the world. The end of the stem is the part of the plant that is most often used in the treatment of depression.

Preparing Saffron involves taking the strands of the plant and either boiling them or grinding them into a powder form. Sprinkle this over your food or you can make yourself a relaxing tea with it.

St. John's Wort. This is a great herb to help battle the throws of depression. St. Johns Wort is grown in North Africa, Europe and Asia. It has been used in the treatment of mild depression in Europe for quite some time now.

It helps to boost the Serotonin levels. Serotonin is known as the body's 'happy chemical' that makes a bond with the neurotransmitters of our brains making us feel good. Many people that are found to suffer from chronic depression often have a chemical imbalance in which they are lacking in this particular chemical. Using a medicinal herb such as St. John's Wort can help to correct this imbalance and get you feeling better in no time.

Chapter 4. Using Medicinal Herbs to Aide in Weight Loss

We have many people around the world that suffer from being overweight. Let us move past all of the fast weight loss gimmicks that are out there and take a look at some natural healthy medicinal herbs that can aide in our weight loss. You may be looking to live a healthier lifestyle or lose some weight whatever the reason there is sure to be a medicinal herb that can help you to reach your personal goals.

Kelp Seaweed. Kelp has been known by the Japanese for many years, as something that could be harvested from the ocean to aide in weight loss. Kelp is very rich in iodine and this can help us with weight loss. It works with your thyroid gland to help give a jump start to your metabolism.

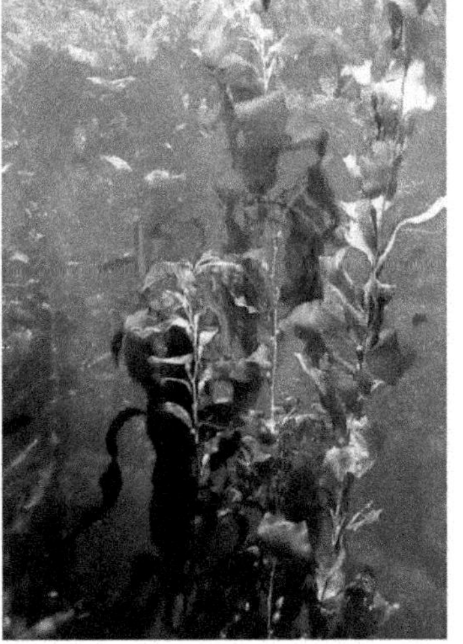

You can ingest it either dried or in a powder form to sprinkle on top of your foods. It has a pretty rich flavor and can be put on many different foods. Using Kelp in soups and salads is one of the more common ways to ingest it. You can buy Kelp at most health food stores and grocery stores.

Gurmar Leaves. Gurmar leaves have been used to treat diabetes and to help aid in weight loss as they are rich in gymnemic acid that is known to help curb the appetite. It will also help to get rid of the cravings for sugar. If you chew on the leaves it can help nullify your sweet tooth for up to six hours.

You might find these leaves very useful if you have a tendency to eat sweets, these leaves can help you to kick eating too many sweets. For thousands of years this has been used in Ayurvedic medicine.

Prickly Pear. The 'Prickly Pear' comes from the cactus family it is found growing in the Mexico area. It has been known to the Native American tribes for a long time and those in Central America as well. It is being used today in treating diabetes, and to help in lowering cholesterol and manage weight loss.

The Prickly Pear is high in antioxidants that tend to help with weight loss. This pear is also used as a cleanser because when it is ingested it helps to reduce the body's water retention and will cleanse the system of excess liquid. This aid in excess water loss will also help in your overall weight loss.

You can find this fruit at most health food stores and it can be grown by private individuals. If you are planning to harvest the plant yourself you should take care and watch out for its thorns. When you purchase it the thorns will be removed already, but if you grow it yourself you will have to remove these sharp little thorns yourself so be careful. It will be a great way for you to improve on your weight loss.

Grapefruit. You may not think of the grapefruit as a medicinal herb, but looks can be deceiving indeed. The grapefruit actually contains a very powerful fat burning molecule that will help your liver to burn up fat rather than storing it. Burning fat rather than storing it is a key factor in successful weight loss regimen.

When having a moderate consumption of grapefruit in your diet it can also help with blood sugar levels by balancing them as well as helping aid in your body's metabolism. It is the juice of the grapefruit that is a great weight loss agent. You could begin your weight loss routine with a glass of grapefruit juice.

Coleus Forskohlii. This is a herb that comes from the mint family, the roots of this medicinal plant contains compounds that can help in boosting your energy while curbing your appetite. Besides aiding in weight loss this herb is also known to help in boosting testosterone in men, it is for this reason that it is often consumed mainly by men.

It is a fact that testosterone helps the body to lose weight and any supplement that increases men's testosterone levels will aid in this task. It is good to boil the root and chop it over salads or used in teas.

Peppermint. Peppermint is a great herb to help with weight loss. It is good for giving you good fresh breath while also aiding in weight loss. The peppermint leaves are packed with properties that help with weight loss.

It also helps to cleanse our systems and can treat digestive problems such as irritable bowel syndrome. Doing this while also raising our level of metabolism and helping to put our body in a state of a healthier weight.

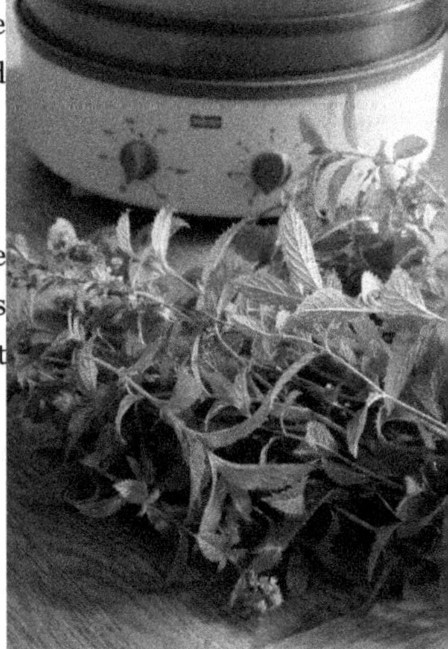

Chapter 5. Wonderful Medicinal Herbs for a Healthy & Long Life

Here in the last chapter of the book we will take a look at the most vital aspect of adding herbal remedies to your life, being able to live a healthy and longer life span. We are all trying to live healthier and longer lives, modern medicine has certainly come along way in helping us to achieve this.

Now many of us are looking towards the ancient past of herbal medicine and what it has to offer in helping us to live healthy and longer lives. Today the maximum human lifespan is in and around 120 years old. There have been people that have been rumoured to live close to 200 years of age—one such man was rumoured to live to be 197 years old.

This man (Li Ching-Yun) was said to live on a diet that consisted of consuming vast amounts of herbs in his daily diet. There is no need to worry you do not have to live on a diet completely made up of medicinal herbs but below are some that you may want to add to your diet.

Rhodiola Rosea.   This amazing herb has been studied extensively by Russian researchers due to its anti-aging properties and healing properties. The properties of this amazing herb have the ability to repair our DNA. It works right at the molecule level to slow down the breakdown of DNA.

Since it is the breakdown of DNA over time that causes us to age, this herb can help us to live longer and better by making sure our DNA works in a healthy way. It also helps raise the immune system and reduces stress, adding yet again more benefits to its anti-aging properties.

Ginkgo Biloba. This is a herb that is well-known in China as the fountain of youth. The tree that it comes from is known to have long longevity with a life span of over 1000 years, this makes them amongst some of the oldest living organisms on this planet.

This wonderful herb helps in restoring, shielding and protecting mitochondria. The mitochondria within our cells is what keeps us functioning properly. The healthy mitochondria are like the foot shoulders of your cell function and are a very fundamental requirement when it come to long and healthy life.

Hawthorn. This medicinal herb is known to have the ability to help strengthen your heart. The most important muscle in your body is your heart. If the heart muscle is not doing a good job at pumping the blood throughout our bodies we are not going to live long.

To live a long and healthy life you must have a healthy heart. People that have had heart failure have added a bit of hawthorn into their diet and have had their hearts strengthened and the previous damage to their hearts repaired.

Chapter 6. Additional Herbal Remedies and How to Prepare and Apply Them

In this final chapter I have added other herbal remedies for common ailments that many of us or loved ones suffer from I hope that you will find them useful and beneficial in aiding with your health needs.

Backache. First you must have your back injury diagnosed to see what is causing your back pain. If it is strained back muscles they will respond to rest, warmth and a treatment of massage. Have your back rubbed two to three times a day with a nice herbal oil or liniment.

You can make an oil by covering St John's Wort herb with olive oil and heating it gently in a pan until it no longer has its fresh green colour and is starting to become crisp. Allow the oil to cool then filter it. Once the oil has been filter it is ready to be applied onto the back with a massage.

Bladder and Urinary Problems. Gravel root is often issued by herbal practitioners to help eliminate urinary buildup in your kidneys. Marshmallow root is also another soothing choice to help with easing the mucous membrane lining of the bladder and urinary system.

Buchu leaves also work well for this type of ailment to be served in a hot infusion it will also soothe pelvic nerves and mucous membranes of the urinary system helping increase the amount of urine secreted. Taking two tablespoonfuls of the infusion three times a day will help in eliminating your urinary infection.

Lowering High Blood Pressure. Garlic is a great herb to use to lower high blood pressure, but will not do your breath a world of good. You can also get it in capsule form. There are also herbal teas that will help lower blood pressure such as hawthorn, lime blossom, nettle or yarrow.

One full glass should be taken three times a day. Your diet should also include lots of leafy greens, raw salads, fresh fruits, onions, and should not include animal fats, alcohol, coffee, and fried foods.

Common Colds and Chills. When you feel chills, sore throat, sneezing these are indications that a cold is developing so take hot infusions of any of these herbs: lemon juice and honey in hot water, peppermint, angelica herb and balm in equal quantities, elderflower and peppermint, yarrow, hyssop and horehound for a chest cold, sage for sore throat take one teaspoonful to half a pint of boiling water, elderflowers and lime blossom taking equal quantities of both when sneezing begins, composition essence take one or two teaspoons to a teacup of hot water for the chills, take plenty of vitamin C between teas on the hour.

Prepare the herbs as infusions that are about the amount of a normal full wineglass.

Constipation. Remedies to help with constipation are:

- Senna Pods: take five or more of them and crush them, adding a pinch of ginger and a cup of boiling water, cover and allow to sit overnight. Drink the liquid once you have strained it in the morning.

- Cascara: You can get it in the form of a liquid extract which you can get from a health food store. Start with a small dose of about five drops in some water at bedtime, increase the dose as needed.

- Linseed: Add a tablespoon of linseed to water and allow it to sit overnight, then add to breakfast cereal to add some bulk to your diet.

- Liquorice root: This is a pleasant tasting laxative, this can be taken alone or added to either senna or cascara to improve their flavour. Peel the sticks before use, add 2 ounces to 2 pints of water and bring to a boil then simmer for ten minutes and strain when it has cooled. Take one wine glass three or more times daily.

Improve your diet by having a whole grain cereal or porridge at breakfast. Add more salads to your diet, stewed prunes which you should eat every day.

Dandruff. Dandruff is related to one's general health. You can take an infusion of nettles taken in one glass full doses to help provide your body with minerals and improve the condition of your scalp; massage your scalp with a lotion that is made from nettles to help stimulate the circulation.

Cut the tops from seeding nettles make sure to wear gloves, shake the tops over a large piece of parchment paper and collect your seeds. Making and infusion with the seeds, boil in water then allow to cool then strain and drink.

Depression. Lavender tea is a good choice to help with depression, it is known as a good nerve tonic; just add three flowering spikes to a cupful of boiling water with a little honey, lavender honey if possible, cover and allow to cool then drink the cool liquid. Ginseng is also a good remedy to help with depression.

You can use powdered Ginseng root, mixing about three ounces of it into a paste using one ounce of honey. Keep this paste in a jar with a screw top lid and take one teaspoonful of this in a cup of boiling water twice daily before your meals. Allow it to stand for ten minutes before you drink it.

The ancient practice of using herbal remedies is becoming more and more sought after in this modern age that we live in.

More people are becoming more interested in the natural solutions to the modern day health problems that they are suffering from. People are being more drawn to the herbal remedies that offer solutions to ailments without a long list of side effects accompanying them like the over the counter prescriptions do.

More and more people are turning away from the synthetic drugs and looking for natural solutions so they can truly be more healthy by taking a natural approach to treating their ailments.

When we apply and use the medicinal herbs that are offered to us in treatment of so many different ailments we can keep ourselves living longer and healthier. We are starting to realize more and more that to better our overall health we need to look into choosing more natural solutions than synthetic ones that always carry side effects with them.

It may take us a bit more effort to prepare the natural choice in medicinal herbal treatments for our ailments but this will certainly be well worth it when we get the positive results that we are seeking from using them. Not only will they be a much healthier form of treatment but they will be much cheaper to purchase compared to the high cost of synthetic medications.

Many of us in our fast paced world go for the quick fix and the convenience of the synthetic medications. Deep down within we all know the best choice is the natural one that is made from materials that contain things that our bodies were meant to ingest unlike synthetic choices that are made up of ingredients that our bodies were not built to ingest.

Conclusion

I hope that you will find the tips and suggestions in my book helpful to you when it comes to you trying to choose some medicinal herbs for your ailments. It is always best to go with a natural choice in most things if you can. I am sure you are going to get the positive results that you seek when you begin to use medicinal herbs to help in treating and possibly curing what ails you.

You will not have to worry about severe side effects as you would when taking synthetic medications. I would suggest talking things over with your doctor and let them know what you would like to do and what medicinal herbs you are interested in trying. It is a good idea to hear the medical opinion of your doctor before you go and make serious changes to the medical treatment you are taking.

Find out the most safe and best way for you to make some changes in your medication choices. It is always best to do your research first before jumping into anything, this way you can make sure that you are well informed and will make some well informed decisions on how you will approach treating your ailments. Whatever you decide I wish you a long and healthy life!

I want to thank you once again for downloading my book I wish you the best of luck in finding the right treatments to help cure or reduce your aches and pains. I hope my suggestions will help you to find some relief or cures of your health issues.

FREE Bonus Reminder

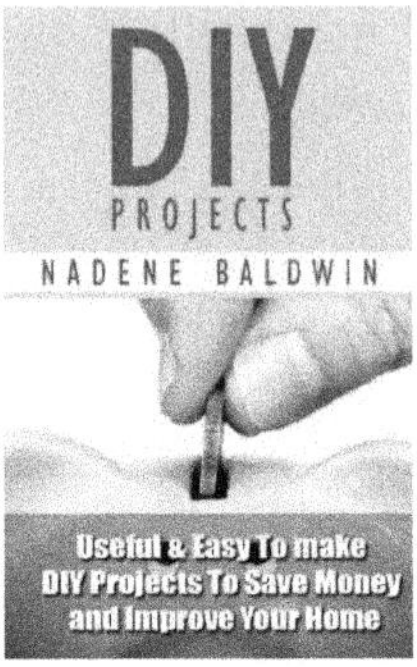

If you have not grabbed it yet, please go ahead and download your special bonus report *"DIY Projects. 13 Useful & Easy To Make DIY Projects To Save Money & Improve Your Home!"*

Simply Click the Button Below

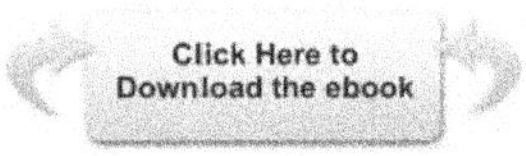

OR **Go to This Page**
http://diyhomecraft.com/free

BONUS #2: More Free & Discounted Books

Do you want to receive more Free & Discounted Books?
We have a mailing list where we send out our new Books when they go free or with a discount on Kindle. Click on the link below to sign up for Free & Discount Book Promotions.

=> Sign Up for Free & Discount Book Promotions <=

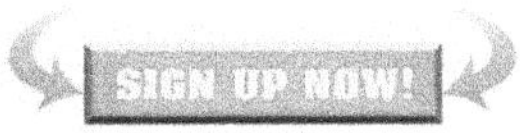

OR Go to this URL
http://zbit.ly/1WBb1Ek